Hajer Nouira
Soumaya Chtioui
Mohamed Fekih Hassen

Méduri protocol and COVID19 pneumonia: Factors in therapeutic failure

Hajer Nouira
Soumaya Chtioui
Mohamed Fekih Hassen

Méduri protocol and COVID19 pneumonia: Factors in therapeutic failure

Predictors of corticosteroid failure in SARS-CoV-2 resuscitation pneumonia

ScienciaScripts

Imprint

Any brand names and product names mentioned in this book are subject to trademark, brand or patent protection and are trademarks or registered trademarks of their respective holders. The use of brand names, product names, common names, trade names, product descriptions etc. even without a particular marking in this work is in no way to be construed to mean that such names may be regarded as unrestricted in respect of trademark and brand protection legislation and could thus be used by anyone.

Cover image: www.ingimage.com

This book is a translation from the original published under ISBN 978-620-6-72043-0.

Publisher:
Sciencia Scripts
is a trademark of
Dodo Books Indian Ocean Ltd. and OmniScriptum S.R.L publishing group

120 High Road, East Finchley, London, N2 9ED, United Kingdom
Str. Armeneasca 28/1, office 1, Chisinau MD-2012, Republic of Moldova, Europe
Printed at: see last page
ISBN: 978-620-8-19061-3

TABLE OF CONTENTS

Introduction 4

Materials and methods 8

Results 15

Discussion 27

Conclusion 37

References 40

Appendices 48

LIST OF ABBREVIATIONS

ACE 2	: Angiotensin-Converting Enzyme *2*
AI	: Aide inspiratoire
APACHE II	: Acute Physiology and chronic Health Evaluation
AVC	: Accident vasculaire cérébral
BPCO	: Broncho-pneumopathie chronique obstructive
Covid-19	: CoronaVirus Disease 2019
CPAP	: Continuous Positive Airway Pressure
CRP	: Protéine C-réactive
Cxcl10	: CXC motif chemokine 10
DV	: Décubitus ventral
ECMO	: Extracorporeal membrane oxygenation
FC	: Fréquence cardiaque
FiO2	: Fraction inspirée en oxygène
FFP2	: Filtering Face Piece
FR	: Fréquence respiratoire
GB	: Globules blancs
HTA	: Hypertension artérielle
IC	: Intervalle de confiance
IFN	: Interféron
IQR	: Interquartile range
IL6	: Interleukine 6
IL-1β	: Interleukine 1β
IL1	: Interleukine 1
IOT	: Intubation oro-trachéale
IV	: *Intra veineux*
MERS-CoV	: Meaddle east respiratory syndrome-*coronavirus*
NF-Kb	: Nuclear factor kappa-light-chain-enhancer of activated B cells
NO	: Monoxyde d'azote
OAP	: Œdème aigu du poumon
OF	: Optiflow

OMS	: Organisation mondiale de santé
OR	: Odds ratio
PaCO2	: Pression artérielle de dioxyde de carbone
PaO2	: Pression artérielle d'oxygène
PAD	: Pression artérielle diastolique
PAS	: Pression artérielle systolique
PEP	: Pression expiratoire positive
PH	: Potentiel hydrogène
ROC	: Receiver Operating Characteristic
RR	: Risque relatif
SAMU	: Service d'aide médicale urgente
SAPS II	: Simplified Acute Physiology Score II
SARS-CoV-1	: Severe acute respiratory syndrome coronavirus 1
SARS-CoV-2	: Severe acute respiratory syndrome coronavirus 2
SAS	: Syndrome d'apnées de sommeil
SDRA	: Syndrome de détresse respiratoire aigu
SOFA	: Sequential Organ Failure Assessment
TDM	: Tomodensitométrie
Test-PCR	: Test Polymerase Chain Reaction
VMI	: Ventilation mécanique invasive
VM	: *Ventilation mécanique*
VNI	: Ventilation non invasive
VPN	: Valeur prédictive négative
VPP	: Valeur prédictive positive
VS	: Versus

INTRODUCTION

INTRODUCTION

Three global health threats secondary to the coronavirus have been observed in less than twenty years (1). Severe acute respiratory syndrome coronavirus 1 (SARS-CoV-1) affected China in 2002. Meaddle east respiratory syndrome-coronavirus (MERS-CoV) was fatal in 2012 in GOLF countries and recently SARS-CoV-2 was identified in Wuhan, China, in 2019. (2). The World Health Organisation has described this latest threat as a pandemic (3).

The SARS-CoV-2 virus binds to angiotensin converting enzyme 2 (ACE 2) to enter the body (4). After an incubation period, 70% of patients will develop dyspnoea, cough and fever (5). The immune response may be inadequate, leading to a worsening of respiratory symptoms, the onset of acute respiratory distress syndrome (ARDS) and an inflammatory reaction (6). This cytokine storm is most often associated with ARDS and viral sepsis (7).

In most cases, the patient has little or no symptoms. Rarely, the condition is severe, leading to ARDS with bilateral involvement (8, 9)shock and death. These symptoms are the result of an uncontrolled immune response and the secretion of cytokines (Interleukin 6 (IL6), Interleukin 1β (IL-1 β), Interferon (IFN) and CXC chemokine motif 10 (cxcl10)) by dendritic cells and macrophages.

Corticoids have anti-inflammatory properties by inhibiting the synthesis of IL-1 and IL-6. They activate the transcription and synthesis of inhibitory Nuclear factor kappa-light-chain-enhancer of activated B cells (NF-Kb) and lipocortin1. They reduce the proliferation, activation and differentiation of T lymphocytes and macrophages (10, 11).

In a meta-analysis including 8 randomised controlled trials with a total of 7737 patients with moderate to severe SARS-CoV-2 pneumonia, 36.1% received Versus (VS) corticosteroid therapy and 63.9% received either a placebo effect or other treatments for pneumonia (other than corticosteroid therapy). (12). Mortality was significantly lower in the corticosteroid group (OR =0.85; CI=95% [0.76-0.95]; p=0.03). Use of mechanical ventilation was significantly reduced in the corticosteroid group (OR=0.76; 95% CI [0.59-0.97]; p=0.03). These results were confirmed by two other meta-analyses (13, 14).

For Chaudhuri et *al.* (13)mortality was significantly lower (RR=0.82; 95% CI [0.72-0.95]).

Chang et *al.* (14) demonstrated that corticosteroid therapy significantly reduces mortality (RR=0.78; CI 95% [0.70-0.87] p < 0.01).

Several types of corticosteroid were used: dexamethasone, hydrocortisone and methylprednisolone. Dexamethasone was compared in three randomised controlled trials: DEXA-COVID 19 (15)CODEX (16)RECOVERY.COM (17). Mortality was significantly reduced in the dexamethasone group (OR=0.64; 95% CI [0.50-0.82]; p < 0.001). However, there was no difference when hydrocortisone or methylprednisolone were used. (18).

In a meta-analysis by Van Paassen et *al.* (19) including 44 studies, methylprednisolone, prednisone, dexamethasone and hydrocortisone were used in 35%, 28%, 5% and 4% respectively. In this study, mortality was reduced (OR=0.72; 95% CI [0.57-0.87]). The number of patients requiring mechanical ventilation was significantly reduced with RR=0.71; 95% CI [0.54-0.97].

The dose of corticosteroids used can be subdivided into "high dose" and "low dose". In the RECOVERY (17)the authors compared two doses: 12 mg dexamethasone versus 6 mg in patients with hypoxemic COVID-19 pneumonia who did not require mechanical ventilation. Mortality was 19% in the high-dose group versus 12% in the low-dose group (RR=1.59; 95% CI [1.2-2.1]; p=0.0012). Side effects of high-dose dexamethasone, such as pneumonia and hyperglycaemia, were significantly more frequent in the high-dose group.

In a meta-analysis, length of stay alive without mechanical ventilation at D28 and D90, mortality at D30 and D90 were reduced in the dexamethasone 6mg group compared with the 12mg group (20).

For Pinzon et *al.* (21)administration of methylprednisolone at a dose ranging from 250-500 mg reduced mortality from 9.5% to 7% and transfer to intensive care from 4.8% to 14%. This result has been confirmed by two meta-analyses (22, 23). However, Si Jing Ton et *al.* (24) found no difference between the "high dose" and the "low dose" in terms of mortality, rate of admission to intensive care, use of mechanical ventilation, duration of mechanical ventilation, incidence of hyperglycaemia and rate of healthcare-associated infections.

The method of administration of corticosteroid therapy has been the subject of several studies (25-27).

For Batirel et *al.* (25)the administration of a bolus corticosteroid reduces the length of stay in intensive care. However, Khokher et *al.* (26) there was no difference in mortality, use of mechanical ventilation or side effects. This result is consistent with the findings of a meta-analysis by Mohanty et *al.* (27).

In our department, all patients with ARDS were treated with dexamethasone at a dose of 6 mg/d, except in the case of fibrosis lesions on computed tomography (CT). In the event of failure, corticosteroid therapy with methylprednisolone at a dose of 2mg/kg/d was administered in four doses. To the best of our knowledge, no studies have identified factors independently associated with the failure of 2mg/kg/d corticosteroid therapy. We thought it would be useful to carry out our study with the aim of identifying factors predictive of corticosteroid failure in SARS-CoV-2 pneumonia.

Materials and Methods

MATERIALS AND METHODS

1. TYPE AND LOCATION OF STUDY :

This is a longitudinal observational and analytical study of the "prospective cohort" type, carried out in the medical intensive care unit of the Taher Sfar Mahdia Hospital over a period of 31 months, between March 2020 and September 2022.

2. STUDY POPULATION :

2.1 INCLUSION CRITERIA :

We included all patients with the following criteria:

* Age over 18.

 *SARS-CoV-2 pneumonia with ARDS criteria according to the 2012 Berlin definition (28) for intubated patients and for other patients the new definitions of ARDS were used (29). SARS-CoV-2 pneumonia was confirmed by a Polymerase Chain Reaction test (Test-PCR).

* Treatment with methylprednisolone at a dose of 2mg/kg/d for more than 7 days.

2.2 NON-INCLUSION CRITERIA :

The patients not included in our study were :

> Patients with a contraindication to corticosteroid therapy: unbalanced diabetes, other active infection, digestive haemorrhage, etc.

> Patients with limited care

2.3 EXCLUSION CRITERIA :

Appearance of a serious side effect of corticosteroid therapy: active digestive haemorrhage, septic shock at the time of the decision to introduce the Meduri protocol, resuscitation delirium or poorly controlled arterial hypertension (AH).

3. STUDY PROTOCOL :

All patients with pneumonia meeting ARDS criteria had a Test-PCR to confirm SARS-CoV-2 infection in addition to oxygen therapy with optiflow (OF) or non-invasive ventilation (NIV), or orotracheal intubation (OTI).

Patients were started on dexamethasone 6mg/d. Corticosteroid therapy at a dose of 2mg/kg/d in 4 doses was prescribed if dexamethasone treatment failed.

Failure is defined as the absence of clinical improvement on day 7 of admission with persistent hypoxaemia with arterial oxygen pressure (PaO2)/inspired oxygen fraction (FiO2) < 250, an alveolar or interstitial syndrome not explained by an infection, or in the case of scanographic lesions favouring progression to pulmonary fibrosis.

Prior to the start of treatment, a bacteriological sample including a tracheal aspiration and/or a cytobacteriological examination of the sputum, a blood culture and a cytobacteriological examination of the urine were taken. If the samples were negative, a dose of 2mg/kg/d was administered daily for 14 days, then 1mg/kg/d for one week, then 0.5mg/kg/d for 3 days, then 0.25mg/kg/d for 3 days, then 0.125mg/kg/d for 3 days.

Failure of corticosteroid therapy (methylprednisolone) is defined by :
- ➢ Lack of clinical improvement (decrease in lung compliance of more than 50% in intubated patients, high oxygen requirements with FiO2 > 70%) after 7 days of treatment.
- ➢ Secondary development of a healthcare-associated infection with or without septic shock
- ➢ Death

During initial management, patients are placed on oxygen therapy with a saturation target of between 90 and 94%. The prone position was used in the event of a PaO2/FiO2 ratio of <150. Preventive, intermediate or curative heparin therapy combined with stress ulcer protection was prescribed. Oral feeding was authorised if FiO2 < 60%. The other patients were given enteral or parenteral nutrition. Antibiotic therapy was prescribed at the start of the pandemic, then in cases of strong suspicion of superinfection or bacterial co-infection. Under corticosteroid therapy, bacteriological samples were taken if superinfection was suspected.

4. PARAMETERS COLLECTED :

The parameters collected were :

4.1 DEMOGRAPHIC CHARACTERISTICS :

- ➢ Age
- ➢ Type

4.2 COMORBIDITIES :

- ➢ Cardiovascular: hypertension, rhythm disorders, ischaemic heart disease
- ➢ Respiratory: asthma, chronic obstructive pulmonary disease (COPD)
- ➢ Metabolic: diabetes, dyslipidaemia

4.3 PATIENT'S REGION :

- ➢ Mahdia
- ➢ Monastir...

4.4 ORIGINAL SERVICE :

- ➢ Emergency
- ➢ Emergency medical service (SAMU)
- ➢ Other hospital department
- ➢ Other hospital

4.5 Long-term treatment

4.6 CLINICAL AND PARACLINICAL DATA :

- ➤ Functional signs: cough, dyspnoea, arthralgia, rhinorrhoea, headache, agueusia, confusion, vomiting, diarrhoea, abdominal pain, etc.

- ➤ Duration of symptoms

- ➤ Length of stay (in the emergency department or in another department) before admission to intensive care

- ➤ Clinical manifestations :

    * Respiratory rate (RR)

    * Heart rate (HR)

    * Temperature

    * Systolic blood pressure

    * Diastolic blood pressure

- ➤ Simplified Acute Physiology Score (SAPS II) at admission (30)This is a score designed to measure the severity of illness in patients admitted to intensive care units. It is calculated from 12 variables over the first 24 hours and ranges from 0 to 163 (appendix 1).

- ➤ Acute Physiology And Chronic Health Evaluation (APACHE II) at admission (31) This is the first generalised severity score to be developed. It is the second version of the Acute Physiology and chronic Health Evaluation. This score is calculated from 12 physiological variables associated with age and a number of pre-existing illnesses. The variables are weighted from 1 to 4 according to their values (appendix 2).

- ➤ Sequential Organ Failure Assessment (SOFA) Inclusion score (32) This score assesses the degree of organ dysfunction. It is made up of six sub-scores: the respiratory system (assessed by the PaO2/FiO2 ratio), the cardiovascular system (assessed by mean arterial pressure, type and dose of vasoactive drugs), the neurological system (assessed by Glasgow score), the renal system (assessed by creatinine or diuresis), liver function (assessed by bilirubin level) and coagulation (assessed by platelet level). Each sub-score is graded from zero to four for a SOFA score ranging from zero to 24 (appendix 3).

- ➢ Severity of ARDS according to the Berlin Classification 2012 (28) in :

    * Minimal: PaO2/FiO2 ratio between 200 and 300

    * Moderate: PaO2/FiO2 ratio between 100 and 200

    * Severe: PaO2/FiO2 ratio less than 100

- ➢ Biological manifestations :

    * PH

    * PaO2

    * Arterial carbon dioxide pressure (PaCO2)

    * Bicarbonate

    * PaO2/FiO2

    * White blood cells

    * Haemoglobin

    * C-reactive protein (CRP)

4.7 THERAPEUTIC MANAGEMENT :

- ➢ Antibiotic therapy
- ➢ Heparin therapy :

    → curative

    → or intermediate

    → or preventive

- ➢ Use of the prone position
- ➢ Oxygen therapy

4.8 PATIENT OUTCOME :

> Response to corticosteroid therapy

> Duration of non-invasive oxygen therapy

> Duration of invasive mechanical ventilation

> Occurrence of healthcare-associated infections :

* Care-associated pneumonia
* blood-vascular infection
* urinary tract infection

> Length of stay in intensive care

> Mortality

5. DATA ENTRY AND ANALYSIS :

They were carried out using SPSS IBM 23 software. Continuous variables are represented by means ± standard deviation. Absolute and relative frequencies were used to express the qualitative variables.

For the univariate analysis, we used the ki2 test to compare two percentages (Fischer's exact test for small numbers) and Student's t test to compare two means. We included in the multivariate analysis all variables with a significance level of less than 20% in the univariate analysis. We then performed a multivariate logistic regression to determine the factors independently associated with treatment failure. The significance level was set at 5%.

A Receiver Operating Characteristic (ROC) curve was performed to identify the threshold that predicts failure of corticosteroid therapy. We also calculated the sensitivity, specificity, positive predictive value (PPV) and negative predictive value (NPV) of these parameters.

RESULTS

RESULTS

1. PATIENT PROFILE :

During the study period, 449 patients were hospitalised with SARS-CoV-2 pneumonia. Of these, 262 were excluded (not taking corticosteroids according to the Meduri protocol). Of the 187 patients included, 9 were excluded secondarily because of a decision to limit care.

A total of 178 patients were included.

1.1 FLOW CHART

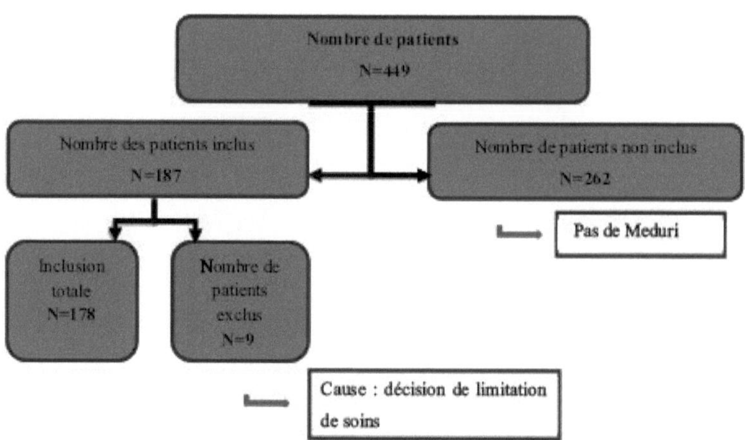

Figure 1: Flow chart of the study

1.2 DEMOGRAPHIC CHARACTERISTICS AND CO-MORBIDITIES :

During the study period, 178 patients with a median age of 62 years in the interquartile range (IQR) [53-68] were included in our study.

Of the patients hospitalised in intensive care, 92% were from the governorate of Mahdia. Emergency departments were the main service of origin for our patients (75%).

The most common co-morbidities were hypertension (43%), diabetes (37%) and dyslipidaemia (19%).

Table I summarises the demographic characteristics, department of origin, co-morbidities and background treatments of patients.

Table I: Demographic characteristics and co-morbidities of patients

	Total population N=178
Age, years (median [IQR])	62 [53-68]
Gender, male n (%)	102(57)
Governorate n (%) :	
Mahdia	164(92)
Monastir	6(3)
Kasserine	2(1)
Other	6(3)
Home department n (%) :	
Emergencies	134(75)
SAMU	8(5)
Transfer from another service	30(17)
Transfer from another hospital	6(9)
Smoking n (%)	30(16)
Comorbidities n (%) :	
SAS	9(5)
Asthma	6(3)
Diabetes	66(37)
HTA	77(43)
Dyslipidemia	33(19)
AVC	8(5)
Chronic renal failure	10(6)
Long-term treatment n (%) :	
Inhaled corticosteroid therapy	6(3)
Oral corticosteroid therapy	35(20)
Insulin therapy	26(15)
Converting enzyme inhibitor	42(24)

IQR: interquartile range, SAMU: emergency medical service, BPCO: chronic obstructive pulmonary disease, SAS: sleep apnoea syndrome, HTA: high blood pressure, AVC: stroke.

1.3 CLINICAL CHARACTERISTICS

The median duration of symptoms was 5 IQR days [3-7].

The most frequent clinical manifestations of SARS-CoV-2 infection were dry cough (53%) and asthenia (51%).

The median SAPS II was 10 IQR [7-13] and the median SOFA score was 4 IQR [3-5].

Severe ARDS was observed in 63% of cases.

Table II illustrates the clinical manifestations observed.

Table II: Clinical characteristics

	Total population N=178
Dry cough, n (%)	94(53)
Rhinorrhoea, n (%)	6(3)
Chest pain, n (%)	10(6)
Asthenia, n (%)	91(51)
Arthralgia, n (%)	30(17)
Agnosia, n (%)	1(1)
Anosmia, n (%)	3(2)
Headache, n (%)	18(10)
Confusion, n (%)	5(3)
Vomiting, n (%)	5(3)
Diarrhoea, n (%)	15(8)
Abdominal pain, n (%)	7(4)
SAPS II; median (IQR)	10[7-13]
APACH II, median (IQR)	27[20-33]
SOFA score, median (IQR)	4[3-5]
Duration of symptoms, n(days)	5[3-7]
Systolic blood pressure (mmHg)	130[120-140]
Diastolic blood pressure (mmHg)	70[70-80]
Heart rate on admission (c/min); median (IQR)	85[75-95]
Respiratory rate on admission (c/min); median (IQR)	28[24-32]
Temperature (°C)	37[37-37]
ARDS n (%) :	
Leger	6(4)
Moderate	59(33)
Severe	112(63)
Length of stay in emergency department, n(days)	2[1-3]

SAPS II: Simplified Acute Physiology Score II, APACHE II: Acute Physiology and chronic Health Evaluation, II, SOFA: Sequential Organ Failure Assessment, ARDS: acute respiratory distress syndrome, IQR: interquartile range

1.4 BIOLOGICAL MANIFESTATIONS :

Table III illustrates the main biological manifestations observed.

The median PaO2 was 78 IQR [64-94] and the median PaO2/FiO2 ratio was 92 IQR [69-143].

Table III: Biological manifestations

	Total population N=178
PH on admission	7,44[7,40-7,47]
PaCO2: mmHg, median IQR	37[32-42]
PaO2: mmHg, median IQR	78[64-94]
Bicarbonates: mmol; median IQR	24[21-27]
PaO2/FiO2	92[69-143]
White blood cells	5431[8102-15192]
Glycated haemoglobin	7,90[6,76-9,37]
CRP	117[77-174]

PH: hydrogen potential, PaCO2: arterial carbon dioxide pressure, IQR: interquartile range, PaO2: arterial oxygen pressure, FiO2: inspiratory fraction of oxygen, CRP: C-reactive protein

1.5 THERAPEUTIC MANAGEMENT AND PROGRESS :

Table IV illustrates patient management and outcomes. Dexamethasone was prescribed in 82% of patients. Only 17% of patients were intubated on admission.

Prone positioning was combined with oxygen therapy in 90% of cases. One hundred and seventeen patients (66%) were responders to prone therapy.

The incidence of nosocomial lung infections was 36%.

Mortality was 61%.

Table IV: Management and progress

	Total population N=178
Dexamethasone	145(82)
Antibiotic	34(19)
Heparin therapy :	
Curative	56(32)
Intermediate	73(41)

Preventive	48(47)
NIV	66(37)
VMI	30(17)
DV	160(90)
Healthcare-associated infections, n (%) :	114(64)
Healthcare-associated lung infection	64(36)
Urinary tract infection	18(10)
Blood-vascular infection	32(18)
NAV duration, n(days)	5(2,25-8)
VMI duration, n(days)	12(6-21,5)
Length of stay, n(days)	14(10-23)
Mortality n (%)	109(61)

NIV: non-invasive ventilation, IMV: invasive mechanical ventilation, VD: prone position

2. ANALYTICAL STUDY: COMPARATIVE STUDY BETWEEN RESPONDERS AND NON-RESPONDERS TO CORTICOSTEROID THERAPY

2.1 UNIVARIATE ANALYSIS

In our study, 60 patients (33.7%) were responders to the Méduri protocol.

In univariate analysis, we found no statistically significant difference in demographic characteristics, comorbidities and long-term treatment between the corticosteroid success group and the failure group.

Table V shows the results for s demographic characteristics, comorbidities and long-term treatment s .

Table V: Demographic characteristics, comorbidities and long-term treatment

	Success Group N=60	Failure group N=118	p

Age ; years	59,5 [52,25-68]	63[55-68]	0,370
Male, n (%)	38(63)	64	0,177
Duration of signs before consultation, median IQR d	1[1-3]	2[1-4]	0,087
Comorbidities, n (%) :			
Asthma	2(3)	4(3)	0,649
Dysthyroidism	2(3)	5(4)	0,575
Diabetes	22(37)	45(38)	0,773
HTA	29(48)	49(41)	0,588
COPD	3(5)	7(6)	0,565
Dyslipidemia	15(25)	19(16)	0,210
Long-term treatment, n (%) :			
Inhaled corticosteroid therapy	2(3)	7(6)	0,377
Oral corticosteroid therapy	12(20)	23(19)	0,783
Insulin therapy	8(13)	19(16)	0,466
Converting enzyme inhibitor	13(22	29(24)	0,730

HTA: high blood pressure, COPD: chronic obstructive pulmonary disease

In univariate analysis, we did not find a statistically significant difference in functional signs and clinical signs between the corticosteroid success group and the failure group.

SAPS II was significantly higher in the failure group: 29 IQR [22-34] versus 21 [17.25-28] p<0.001. The median APACHE II score was 10 [8-14] in the failure group versus 7 [6-10] in the success group p<0.001.

Table VI: Functional signs, clinical signs and biological manifestations

	Success Group N=60	Failure group N=118	p
Clinical signs, n (%) :			
Dry cough	32(53)	63(53)	0,960
Rhinorrhea	1(2)	5(4)	0,351
Dyspnoea	52(87)	102(86)	0,896
Fever	30(50)	55(46))	0,561
Chest pain	3(5)	7(6)	0,565
Asthenia	32(55)	59(50)	0,558
Arthralgia	11(18)	19(16)	0,653

Headaches	5(8)	13(11)	0,610
Oxygen therapy, n (%) :			
Invasive	2(3)	28(24)	<0,001
OF	54(90)	95(80)	0,105
Non-invasive	17(28)	50(42)	0,034
Prone, n (%)	52(87)	108(91)	0,585
Severity of ARDS :			
Leger	2(3)	4(4)	1,000
Moderate	26(43)	33(28)	0,003
Severe	32(54)	82(69)	0,014
SAPS II, median IQR	21[17-28]	29[22-34]	<0,001
APACH II, median IQR	7[6-10]	10[8-14]	<0,001
SOFA, median IQR	4[3-4]	4[4-5]	0,121
PAS (mmHg)	130[120-150]	130[120-140]	0,127
DBP (mmHg)	80[70-80]	30[26-34]	0,273
PH	7,44[7,41-7,48]	7,43[7,38-7,47]	0,181
PaCO2 admission, median IQR	37,5[33-40]	36[31-42]	0,652
PaO2 admission, median IQR	79,5[66,25-98,5]	77[64-92]	0,903
PaO2/FiO2, median IQR	102[79,50-154,75]	86[69-127]	0,031
GB, median IQR	11600[8925-14800]	11000[7550-16100]	0,604
Lymphocytes, median IQR	800[525-940]	700[520-990]	0,635

OF: OptiFlow, ARDS: acute respiratory distress syndrome, SAPS II: Simplified Acute Physiology Score, IQR: interquartile range, APACHE II Score: Acute Physiology and chronic Health Evaluation, SOFA: Sequential Organ Failure Assessment, PAS: systolic blood pressure, DBP: diastolic blood pressure, PH: hydrogen potential, PaCO2: arterial carbon dioxide pressure, PaO2: arterial oxygen pressure, FiO2: inspiratory fraction of oxygen, WBC: white blood cells.

There was no significant difference in the antibiotic therapy prescribed on admission (24% vs 8%) p=0.09 and curative dose heparin therapy (40% vs 13%) < 0.001 in favour of the failure group.

Progression was marked by a significantly higher incidence of complications in the failure group. This concerns the rates of nosocomial infections 35% VS 79%.

p= 0.037, barotrauma 3% VS 24% p < 0.001 and acute renal failure 5% VS 31% p < 0.001.

Table VII illustrates the biological manifestations, management and evolution of the disease.

Table VII: Patient management and outcome

	Success Group N=60	Failure group N=118	p
Antibiotic therapy, n (%)	5[8]	29[24]	0,009
Heparin therapy, n (%) :			
Curative	8[13]	48[40]	<0,001
Intermediate	31[52]	43[36]	0,051
Preventive	21[35]	27[24]	0,072
Progression to fibrosis, n (%)	4[7]	15[13]	0,217
Healthcare-associated infections, n (%)	21[35]	94[79]	0,037
Complications, n (%) :			
Barotrauma	2[3]	29[24]	<0,001
Renal insufficiency	3[5]	37[31]	<0,001
Hyperglycaemia	3[5]	11[9]	0,310
Thromboembolic	4[7]	5[4]	0,481
Time from admission to IOT, D median IQR	1[0-1]	5,73[2-8]	<0.001
Duration of sedation, median D IQR	7,5[4-13,25]	12[6-20]	0,356
Curarisation time, median J IQR	5,5[1,25-10,50]	10[5-17]	0,420
VMI duration, D median IQR	8[0-22]	12,5[6-21,75]	0,352
NIV duration, D median IQR	7,06[3,50-10,25]	4[2-7,25]	0,173
Length of stay in intensive care, median IQR J	11[9-16]	17[11,75-26,25]	
Mortality, n (%)	0(0)	109[91,6]	<0,001

OTI: orotracheal intubation, IMV: invasive mechanical ventilation, NIV: non-invasive ventilation

As regards ventilatory management of patients, there was a significant difference in the invasive and non-invasive oxygen therapy used. In fact, only 3% of patients in the success group were ventilated invasively compared with 24% in the failure group (p<0.001), while NIV was prescribed in 28% of the success group compared with 42% in the failure group (p=0.034). There was no difference in the prescribed parameters of mechanical ventilation, whether invasive or non-invasive.

Table VIII illustrates the parameters of invasive and non-invasive ventilation.

Table VIII: Non-invasive and invasive ventilation parameters

	Successful N=60	Failure N=118	p
High-flow oxygen therapy, Flow of o₂	60L/m² of water	60L/m	0,999
Non-invasive ventilation			
PEP	6[6-8]	8[6-8]	0,244
AI	10[8-12]	10[8-12]	0,271
Invasive mechanical ventilation			
Tidal volume ml/Kg	400[385-415]	420[380-447]	0,771
FR	28[25-29,5]	30[28-32]	0,716
PEP	11[8,5-13,5]	10[28-32]	0,150
Platen pressure	23,5[17,5-31]	29[26-30]	0,017
Driving pressure	14,5[11-17,5]	17[14.25-21]	0,211
Lung compliance	28,5[24,25-45,50]	23[18-29]	0,019

PEP: positive expiratory pressure, AI: inspiratory aid, FR: respiratory frequency

Table IX shows the evolution of white blood cells, CRP and certain ventilatory parameters. The white blood cell count was similar between the two groups from D1 to D28. However, there was a statistically significant difference in CRP values at D3 and D7 between the success and failure groups, in favour of the failure group.

The PaO2/FiO2 ratio was significantly higher between D7 and D14 in favour of the success group 126 [88-175.5] vs 100 [83-125.5] p=0.006 at D3, and 188 [171-297] vs 122 [73-158] p=0.001 at D7.

Changes in tidal volume, positive expiratory pressure (PEEP), motor pressure and lung compliance were similar between the two groups.

Table IX: Changes in ventilatory and biological parameters up to D28

	Success Group	Failure group	p
Leukocytes (10³/µL), median IQR			
Admission	11,6[8,9-14,8]	11[7,5-16,1]	0,665
J1	11,6[8,87-16,70]	12,67[8,9-16,5]	0,661
J3	126[8,4-13,8]	13,6[10,2-18,6]	0,103
J7	19,3[13,2-24,6]	15,6[11,1-20]	0,053
J14	12,7[10,2-19,4]	14,9[11,5-20,7]	0,520
J21	8,9[7,2-16]	13,5[8,5-19,8]	0,424
J28	7[4,8-7]	15,5[13,2-22,3]	0,049
CRP (mg/L), median IQR			
J1	104[66,75-150]	118[67-178]	0,280
J3	31[16,5-94,5]	93[36-145]	<0,001
J7	29[8-77]	123[53-199]	<0,001
J14	16[7,5-105,5]	73[24-173]	0,076
J21	77[49-85]	87,5[29,5-175]	0,241
J28	65[4-143]	131[76-170]	0,186
Tidal volume (ml/Kg), median IQR			
J1	400[400-400]	440[400-460]	0,259
J3	410(400-420)	430[400-460]	0,614
J7	410[400-420]	440[400-480]	0,541
J14		420[400-480]	
J21		440[420-495]	
J28		460[425-478]	
Driving pressure (cmH₂O)			
Admission		17,73[14,25-21]	
J1	15[4-15]	16[14,75-21]	0,540
J3	12,5[12-12,5]	17[15-21]	0,230
J7	13[13-13]	18,5[15-22,5]	0,330
J14		21[16,5-22]	
J21		22[18-24]	
J28		26[25-32,5]	
PaO2/FiO2			
Admission		78[66-55]	
J1	122[66-148]	98[69-159]	0,959
J3	116[87-157]	102[81,75-147]	0,465
J7	126[88-175,5]	100[83-125,5]	0,006
J14	188[171-297]	122[73-158]	0,001
J21	195[129-279]	130[81,75-176]	0,113
J28		178[95-228]	
PEP (cmH₂O)			
J1	7[4,5-12]	10[9,5-12]	0,103
J3	6[4-6]	10[6,5-12]	0,382
J7	6[3-6]	10[8-12]	0,168
J14	6[3-6]	8[6-10,5]	0,494
J21		6[6-9]	
J28		4[2-4]	
Lung compliance (ml/cmH₂O)			
J1	29[7-29]	29[21-32]	0,871
J3	26,5[5-26,5]	26[19,5-30,5]	0,940
J7	32[32-32]	21,5[19,5-30,5]	0,363
J14		18[16-26]	
J21		19[15-29]	
J28		18,50[13,75-26]	

CRP: C-reactive protein, PaO2: arterial oxygen pressure, FiO2: inspiratory oxygen fraction PEP: positive expiratory pressure

2.2 MULTIVARIATE ANALYSIS :

In multivariate analysis, the factors independently associated with failure of corticosteroid therapy were the SAPS II severity score OR=0.938; 95% CI [0.895-0.982] p=0.007, and the use of non-invasive mechanical ventilation with OR=0.416; 95% CI [0.187-0.925] p=0.031.

Table X shows the factors independently associated with the failure of corticosteroid therapy.

Table X: Factors independently associated with failure of corticosteroid therapy

Factors	OR	95% CI	p
SAPS II	0,938	[0,895-0,982]	0,007
SOFA	0,737	[0,484-1,122]	0,154
Severity of ARDS	1,641	[0,462-5,829]	0,443
Invasive mechanical ventilation	0,115	[0,013-1,025]	0,053
Non-invasive ventilation	0,416	[0,187-0,925]	0,031
PaO_2/FiO_2 on admission	1,005	[0,990-1,020]	0,547

SAPS II: Simplified Acute Physiology Score II, SOFA: Sequential Organ Failure Assessment, ARDS: acute respiratory distress syndrome,

The threshold value for SAPS II was around 23.5, with a sensitivity of 75% and a specificity of 61%. The zone was 0.724, PPV=54.55 and NPV=79.46 (Figure 2).

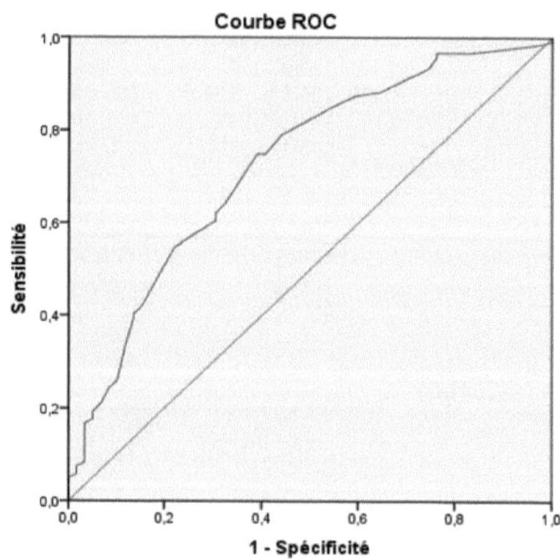

Figure 2: ROC curve for SAPS II score and threshold value

DISCUSSION

DISCUSSION

SARS-CoV-2 infection is a multi-systemic disease, characterised by hyperactivation of coagulation with hypo-fibrinolysis.

In SARS-CoV-2 infection, the initial immune response is ineffective, leading to an amplification of the inflammatory response. This excessive response, which exceeds regulation, leads to clinical worsening, generally on the eighth day after infection and onset of symptoms. Pulmonary involvement may progress to ARDS and multi-visceral failure with signs of immune system hyperactivation (33).

The primary role of corticosteroid therapy is to counteract the excessive inflammatory reaction and the cytokine storm.

In our study, 33.7% of patients responded to high-dose corticosteroid therapy according to the Méduri protocol. We found two factors independently associated with steroid failure: use of NIV and a SAPS score >23.5.

The Covid 19 virus infects pneumocytes expressing ACE 2 (34) and consequently between 67 and 85% of patients admitted to the intensive care unit will develop ARDS (6). The virus also infects cells in the digestive tract which express ACE 2 receptors, in particular enterocytes (35, 36). The disease is characterised by a frequently observed cytolytic disorder and the rarity of cholestatic jaundice (5, 37, 38).

Since ACE 2 is poorly represented in the brain, other hypotheses have been put forward involving nicotinic acetylcholine receptors in the genesis of brain invasion. (39). The neurological tropism of SARS-CoV-2 explains the agueusia, anosmia, muscle damage and damage to the medullary respiratory centre (40). In our study, agueusia, anosmia, headache and confusional syndromes were observed in 1%, 3%, 18% and 5% respectively.

ACE 2 is expressed in tubular cells and to a lesser extent in glomerular cells. Renal involvement is not rare. It can occur in between 5 and 20% of cases (41). In our study, renal failure was rarely observed on admission but was frequent during the course of the disease.

ACE 2 is also expressed by myocardial cells, which explains the presence of several cases of myocarditis. Heart failure is observed in between 7 and 20% of cases (42-44) and 1% of hospitalised patients have an increase in troponins (45). In our study, no cases of myocarditis or heart failure were observed.

Several studies have investigated the value of corticosteroid therapy in the management of SARS-CoV-2pneumonia. Most of these studies were conducted in medical wards and were retrospective and/or observational. They used corticosteroid therapy at a dose $\geq$ 1mg/kg/d at an early stage and for a limited duration, generally less than 10 days.

Three studies have been carried out in intensive care. Nelson et *al.* (46)administration of methylprednisolone at a dose $\geq$ 1mg/kg after disease progression < 14 days resulted in a significant improvement in a composite which included the number of days living without mechanical ventilation and the extubation rate.

In a multicentre randomised controlled trial including 299 patients with moderate or severe ARDS, administration of dexamethasone at a dose of 20 mg/d for 5 days followed by 10 mg intravenously (IV) for 5 days or at discharge was associated with a reduction in survival and survival alive without mechanical ventilation at D28 (16).

In the study by Lu Chen (47)the authors demonstrated an increase in organ failure in the control group, but no difference in mortality.

Table XI shows the results of the main studies using high-dose corticosteroids in the treatment of SARS-CoV-2 pneumonia.

Table XI: Results of the main studies using high-dose corticosteroids in the treatment of SARS-CoV-2 pneumonia

AUTHOR	REFERENCE	PROTOCOL	SAMPLE SIZE	TYPE OF STUDY	RESULTS
Bani-Sadr	(48)	1mg/kg methylprednisolone or 0.5mg/kg if ritonavir Duration= 2 to 3 weeks early	-85 before (no corticosteroids) -172 after -inpatients	Cohort with a historical group	-Reduced mortality in the "after" period RR=0.47; reduced number of intensive care unit admissions and deaths.
Fadel	(49)	Methylprednisolone 0.5-1mg/kg in 2 doses over 3 days for intensive care patients It lasts 7 days.	213 patients with moderate to severe disease	Quasi-experimental	-Reduction in mortality 26.3% VS 21.7%; p=0.024 -Use of VM: 36.6 days VS 21.7 days p=0.025 -Admission to intensive care 44.3% VS 27.3%; p=0.017
Fernandez	(50)	Methylprednisolone 1-2mg/kg for 3 to 5 days	463 Moderate and severe ARDS + hyperinflammation	Retrospective	-Reduction in mortality 13.9% VS 23.9 - No difference between boli and discontinuous administration
Gong Guan	(51)	Methylprednisolone > 1mg/kg for 10 days	-34 patients -Age < 54 in emergency	Retrospective - observational	- Improvements in symptoms, oxygenation and disease progression
Hu Wang	(52)	Prednisolone or methylprednisolone between 0.75-1.5mg/kg/d	308 patients hospitalised	Retrospective - observational	-No effect

Li Zhou	(53)	Methylprednisolone 0.75-1.5 mg/kg/d for 3 days then prednisolone 40-80mg Duration of treatment < 7 days	187 Radiological worsening	Retrospective - observational	-Reduction in the use of VM: 45 VS 74.2
Luchen	(47)	Methylprednisolone 1.5mg/d or dexamethasone 1.25mg/d Median duration 8 days	244:ARDS (PaO2/FiO2< 300) or (Spo$_2$/FiO2<315) or sepsis +organ failure	Retrospective - observational	-Increase in organ failure -No difference in mortality
Ma Zeng	(54)	Methylprednisolone 1-2mg/kg for 3-5 days	450 severe and non-severe	Multicentre retrospective observational	-The length of stay in the corticosteroid group was similar to that in the placebo group.

(Table X continued)

AUTHOR	REFERENCE	PROTOCOL	SAMPLE SIZE	TYPE OF STUDY	RESULTS
Majmundar .M et al	(55)	Prednisolone, dexamethasone methylprednisolone ≥ 1mg/kg	205 patients on the medical ward	Retrospective - observational	-Reduction of the composite (transfer and/or intubation and/or VM
Mikulska et al	(56)	Methylprednisolone ≥ 1mg/kg/d	215 non-intubated patients	Retrospective - observational	-Combination of corticosteroids and tocilizumab improves prognosis
Nelson et al	(46)	Methylprednisolone ≥1mg/kg < 14 days maintenance	117 VM	Retrospective - observational	-Increase in the number of days without VM and the extubation rate
Francisco Salton et al	(57)	80 mg methylprednisolone bolus then 80mg/d	173 ARDS	Retrospective - observational	Composite: death and or transfer to intensive

| | | for 08 days until PaO2/FiO2>350 or CRP<20mg/l then 16mg or 20mg/d IV to achieve CRP<20mg/l and P/F>400 | | | care or use of VM (22.9% VS 44.4%) |
| **Tamazini** | (16) | 20mg/d for 05d then10mg/d IV for 05d until discharge | 299: Moderate or severe ARDS | Multicentre randomised controlled trial | Composite: follow-up at D28 and VM-free survival at D28 In favour of controlled group |

MV: mechanical ventilation, ARDS: acute respiratory distress syndrome, Pao2: arterial oxygen pressure, Fio2: inspiratory oxygen fraction, Spo2: pulsed O2 saturation, CRP: C-reactive protein

Our study was distinguished by a different protocol. We used high-dose corticosteroids after failure of low-dose corticosteroids and/or when early fibrosis lesions appeared. Furthermore, the administration of corticosteroids in our study was a rescue prescription, as it was the only hope of saving our patients given the unavailability of circulatory assistance such as extracorporeal membrane oxygenation (ECMO). In our study, 33.7% of patients were discharged alive after administration of high-dose corticosteroids.

The two factors independently associated with failure were: the SAPS II score with a threshold value of 23.5 and the prescription of non-invasive ventilation.

Our results cannot be compared with other studies since, to the best of our knowledge, there are no published studies on the effect of late administration of a high dose of corticosteroids.

The beneficial effect of the combination of NIV and corticosteroids is explained by the physiological and clinical effect of NIV. The use of NIV in patients with de novo acute respiratory failure other than acute pulmonary oedema (AOP) is controversial. At the start of the pandemic, the use of NIV was exceptional, due to the fear of viral particles being sprayed. Some studies have shown that NIV can be a good alternative to invasive mechanical ventilation. NIV improves muscle work and oxygenation, and reduces the need for invasive mechanical ventilation, not to mention reducing the number of infectious episodes. In our study, 79% of patients had failed corticosteroid therapy compared with 35% in the success group (p=0.037). Although NIV was used in 48% of patients in the failure group compared with 28% in the success group (p=0.034), the failure rate was higher, as shown by the duration of NIV (7.06 [3.5-10.25] vs. 4 [2-7.25]), indicating early failure of NIV.

The beneficial effect of NIV also involves improving oxygenation.

The pH at admission was similar between the two groups, as was the PaO2/FiO2 ratio. However, in the multivariate analysis, there was a significant improvement in the ratio at D7 and D14. This improvement may be due to the application of NIV. It should be noted that our challenge in prescribing NIV parameters was to avoid over-distension caused by the use of excessive inspiratory aids, thus generating high tidal volumes and a source of ventilation-induced lesions (VILI).

The second result obtained concerns the SAPS II score and its threshold value of 23.5. We were persuaded that the most severe patients respond poorly to corticosteroid therapy. Several parameters testify to this severity, such as more frequent recourse to invasive mechanical ventilation (3% VS 24%, p<0.001), the frequency of severe ARDS (54% VS 69%, p=0.014) and a median PaO2/FiO2 ratio of 102 IQR [79.50-154.75] VS 86 IQR [69-127]. In the absence of other therapeutic alternatives, the use of corticosteroids was a necessity in this endemic setting.

With regard to corticosteroid therapy and mortality, although mortality was zero in the success group, it was almost certain (91.6%) in the failure group. In fact, patients who did not respond to corticosteroid therapy were exposed to complications of intensive care, with exposure to nosocomial infections (35% vs. 79%, p=0.037), barotrauma (5% vs. 31%, p<0.001), which is a direct indicator of the severity of pulmonary lesions, and an increase in the length of stay in intensive care.

Unlike SARS in 2003, which was responsible for a variable mortality rate of between 13 and 64% (58-61)SARS-CoV-2 was more fatal. Mortality was 69% in China and 73% in Poland (62). This mortality rate concerns all patients hospitalised for management of SARS-CoV-2 pneumonia. Furthermore, the mortality observed in our study is in line with international standards.

Concerning corticosteroid therapy and CRP: the aim of late corticosteroid therapy is to prevent progression to pulmonary fibrosis and refractory hypoxaemia. Although corticosteroid therapy was prescribed late compared with the studies, we noted that CRP was elevated in both groups from the first days 104 [66.75-150] in the success group compared with 118 [67-178] in the failure group. This indicates the existence of a pre-existing inflammatory syndrome beyond 10 days. CRP levels at D3 and D7 were significantly lower in the success group than in the failure group. However, this difference disappeared during the course of the treatment, probably indicating the existence of other causes of inflammatory reactions, such as hospital-acquired infections. It should be noted that Francisco Salton et *al.*, in a retrospective observational study including 173 patients with ARDS, prescribed corticosteroids on the basis of CRP values. Their protocol consisted of administering a bolus of 80mg then 80mg/d for 8 days until a PaO2/FiO2 ratio ≥ 350 or a CRP < 20mg/l then 16 or 20 mg/d IV to achieve a CRP < 20mg/l and PaO2/FiO2 ≥ 400. In this study, the endpoint was a composite (mortality and/or use of mechanical ventilation). The composite was significantly reduced from 22.9% to 44.4%.

Corticosteroids and effect on ventilatory parameters: In our study, motor pressure from D1 to D28, positive expiratory pressure from D1 to D28, tidal volume from D1 to D28 and lung compliance from D1 to D28 were identical between the two groups and there was no statistically significant difference. Our ventilatory management of ARDS secondary to SARS-CoV-2 infection follows international recommendations (63). The primary objective of this management is to prevent mechanical ventilation-induced injury by using a reduced tidal volume ≤ 6 ml/kg and a PEEP to have a plateau pressure ≤ 30cmH2O. Analysis of these findings leads to this conclusion: the success of corticosteroid therapy did not influence ventilatory parameters, so its effectiveness is determined by the improvement in the PaO2/FiO2 ratio. This leads us to conclude that early evaluation of corticosteroid therapy should probably take into account the PaO2/FiO2 ratio rather than plateau pressure and pulmonary compliance. In fact, in the success group, pulmonary compliance increased from 29 [7-29] at D1 to 32 [32-32] at D7. Whereas pulmonary compliance fell from 23 [18-29] to 18.5 [13.75-26] in the failure group. I believe that these findings should be taken into account to minimise the deleterious effects of corticosteroid therapy and to stop it before the patient develops infectious, metabolic and peripheral neurological complications in the event of no improvement in PaO2/FiO2 and pulmonary compliance at D7.

Our study is most likely the first to evaluate the prescription of high-dose late corticosteroids in the management of ARDS secondary to SARS-CoV-2 pneumonia.

Our study has a number of limitations. On the one hand, it is a prospective, non-randomised observational cohort study.

The absence of randomisation is a bias which may have an impact on the results obtained. Our decision to prescribe corticosteroids was a matter of absolute necessity and rescue in the absence of other available therapeutic means, so randomisation was not possible.

On the other hand, it is a mono-centric study carried out in the medical intensive care unit of the Taher Sfar hospital in Mahdia.

The enrichment of our results by the experience of other departments is very interesting since, on the one hand, we will have a larger sample, thus avoiding certain biases and, on the other hand, therapeutic management with other therapeutic means (ECMO, ECALTA, antivirals) associated with corticosteroid therapy could improve survival. In fact, our management was appropriate and in line with international recommendations, particularly in terms of oxygen therapy, prescription of ventilatory parameters, administration of corticosteroids, heparin therapy, use of the prone position and nitric oxide. The only difference was that ECMO was not used in severe cases. This technique was not available in several departments and is rarely used due to technical difficulties.

In addition, the size of the sample may be at the origin of a type 2 error. We believe that our sample is acceptable since it concerns intensive care patients.

In the light of our study, a number of recommendations can be made:

- Use of preventive measures Filtering Face Piece (FFP2), hand washing, isolation, etc.
- Use of oxygen therapy adapted to each case, favouring non-invasive methods, essentially high-flow oxygen therapy, NIV and CPAP.
- For ventilated patients, mechanical ventilation-induced injury should be prevented by using a tidal volume $\leq$ 6ml/kg and adequate PEEP to achieve a plateau pressure $\leq$ 30 CmH2O
- In the event of PaO2/FiO2 < 150, the patient should be placed in the prone position with or without vigour.

- If there is no improvement, the use of NO (nitric oxide) should be discussed on a case-by-case basis.
- Severe forms require circulatory assistance via ECMO.
- Corticosteroids should be prescribed early, at a dose of 10mg/d for 10 days. If there is no improvement, or if the disease is progressing towards incipient pulmonary fibrosis, high-dose corticosteroids should be used, with a follow-up on day 7 to assess efficacy and decide whether or not to continue corticosteroids.
- Heparin therapy should be used as indicated at an intermediate dose.
- No systematic indication for antibiotic therapy.

CONCLUSION

CONCLUSION

The WHO has described coronavirus disease as a pandemic. Mortality in intensive care has exceeded 60%. SARS-CoV-2 is characterised by an excessive inflammatory reaction and a cytokine storm. The anti-inflammatory effects of corticosteroids have been shown to be effective in reducing mortality in severe patients with ARDS. Most studies have investigated the efficacy of corticosteroids in the early phase of lung damage, but the inflammatory reaction may last for more than 8 days . In addition, some patients are managed late for various reasons, the initial corticosteroid therapy fails and the disease progresses to pulmonary fibrosis. In this context, we conducted this study to determine the factors independently associated with the failure of high-dose corticosteroid therapy.

We carried out a prospective cohort and analytical study including all patients hospitalised for the management of SARS-CoV-2 pneumonia and treated with corticosteroid therapy according to the Meduri protocol, which consists of starting patients on methylprednisolone at a dose of 2mg/kg/d administered daily for 14 days, then 1mg/kg/d for one week, then 0.5mg/kg/d for 3 days, then 0.25mg/kg/d for 3 days, then 0.125mg/kg/d for 3 days.

We analysed demographic parameters, comorbidities, functional, clinical and paraclinical manifestations, the severity of the clinical picture by calculating two severity scores (SAPS II and APACHE II), the organ failure score (SOFA) and the severity of ARDS, ventilatory parameters: type of oxygen therapy with parameters used, monitoring parameters (compliance, motor pressure), complications of corticosteroid therapy: nosocomial infections, hyperglycaemia, complications of mechanical ventilation: pneumopathy associated with mechanical ventilation, barotrauma, length of stay, duration of mechanical ventilation and mortality.

During the study period 178 patients with a median age of 62 years [53-68] were included.

The most common comorbidities were hypertension (43%) and diabetes (37%). The median time to onset of symptoms was 5 days [3-7]. Severe ARDS was present in 63% of cases.

Mortality was 61%. The success rate of corticosteroid therapy was 33.7%.

In multivariate analysis, SAPS II (OR=0.938; CI95% [0.895-0.982] p=0.007) and use of non-invasive ventilation (OR=0.416; CI95% [0.187-0.925] p=0.031) were the factors independently associated with failure of corticosteroid therapy. The SAPS II cut-off value was 23.5 with a sensitivity of 75%, a specificity of 61%, a positive predictive value of 54.55%, a negative predictive value of 79.46% and a zone of 0.724.

In conclusion, 33.7% of patients responded to high-dose corticosteroid therapy after failure of initial corticosteroid therapy. Patients treated with NIV and/or with SAPS II < 23.5 may be candidates for this protocol.

REFERENCES

REFERENCES

1   Wong G, Liu W, Liu Y, Zhou B, Bi Y, Gao GF. MERS, SARS, and Ebola: The Role of Super-Spreaders in Infectious Disease. Cell Host Microbe. 2015;18(4):398-401.

2.   Zhu N, Zhang D, Wang W, Li X, Yang B, Song J, et al. A Novel Coronavirus from Patients with Pneumonia in China, 2019. N Engl J Med. 2020;382(8):727-33.

3   Ye Z, Wang Y, Colunga-Lozano LE, Prasad M, Tangamornsuksan W, Rochwerg B, et al. Efficacy and safety of corticosteroids in COVID-19 based on evidence for COVID-19, other coronavirus infections, influenza, community-acquired pneumonia and acute respiratory distress syndrome: a systematic review and meta-analysis. CMAJ. 2020 Jul 6;192(27):E756-E767. doi:10.1503/cmaj.200645. Epub 2020 May 14. PMID: 32409522; PMCID: PMC7828900.

4   Zhou P, Yang XL, Wang XG, Hu B, Zhang L, Zhang W, et al. A pneumonia outbreak associated with a new coronavirus of probable bat origin. Nature. 2020;579(7798):270-3.

5.   Guan WJ, Ni ZY, Hu Y, Liang WH, Ou CQ, He JX, et al. Clinical Characteristics of Coronavirus Disease 2019 in China. N Engl J Med. 2020;382(18):1708-20.

6   Huang C, Wang Y, Li X, Ren L, Zhao J, Hu Y, et al. Clinical features of patients infected with 2019 novel coronavirus in Wuhan, China. Lancet. 2020;395(10223):497-506.

7   Li H, Liu L, Zhang D, Xu J, Dai H, Tang N, et al. SARS-CoV-2 and viral sepsis: observations and hypotheses. Lancet. 2020;395(10235):1517-20.

8   Dastan F, Saffaei A, Mortazavi SM, Jamaati H, Adnani N, Samiee Roudi S, et al. Continues renal replacement therapy (CRRT) with disposable hemoperfusion cartridge: A promising option for severe COVID-19. J Glob Antimicrob Resist. 2020;21:340-1.

9   Jamaati H, Dastan F, Tabarsi P, Marjani M, Saffaei A, Hashemian SM. A Fourteen-day Experience with Coronavirus Disease 2019 (COVID-19) Induced Acute Respiratory Distress Syndrome (ARDS): An Iranian Treatment Protocol. Iran J Pharm Res. 2020;19(1):31-6.

10. Masjedi M, Esmaeil N, Saffaei A, Abtahi-Naeini B, Pourazizi M, Haghjooy Javanmard S, et al. Cytokine Indexes in Pemphigus Vulgaris: Perception of Its Immunpathogenesis and Hopes for Non-Steroidal Treatment. Iran J Pharm Res. 2017;16(3):1223-9.

11 Rhen T, Cidlowski JA. Antiinflammatory action of glucocorticoids--new mechanisms for old drugs. N Engl J Med. 2005;353(16):1711-23.

12. Pulakurthi YS, Pederson JM, Saravu K, Gupta N, Balasubramanian P, Kamrowski S, et al. Corticosteroid therapy for COVID-19: A systematic review and meta-analysis of randomized controlled trials. Medicine (Baltimore). 2021;100(20):e25719.

13. Chaudhuri D, Sasaki K, Karkar A, Sharif S, Lewis K, Mammen MJ, et al. Corticosteroids in COVID-19 and non-COVID-19 ARDS: a systematic review and meta-analysis. Intensive Care Med. 2021;47(5):521-37.

14 Chang X, Li S, Fu Y, Dang H, Liu C. Safety and efficacy of corticosteroids in ARDS patients: a systematic review and meta-analysis of RCT data. Respir Res. 2022;23(1):301.

15 Villar J, Anon JM, Ferrando C, Aguilar G, Munoz T, Ferreres J, et al. Efficacy of dexamethasone treatment for patients with the acute respiratory distress syndrome caused by COVID-19: study protocol for a randomized controlled superiority trial. Trials. 2020;21(1):717.

16 Tomazini BM, Maia IS, Cavalcanti AB, Berwanger O, Rosa RG, Veiga VC, et al. Effect of Dexamethasone on Days Alive and Ventilator-Free in Patients With Moderate or Severe Acute Respiratory Distress Syndrome and COVID-19: The CoDEX Randomized Clinical Trial. JAMA. 2020;324(13):1307-16.

17. Group RC, Horby P, Lim WS, Emberson JR, Mafham M, Bell JL, et al. Dexamethasone in Hospitalized Patients with Covid-19. N Engl J Med. 2021;384(8):693-704.

18. Group WHOREAfC-TW, Sterne JAC, Murthy S, Diaz JV, Slutsky AS, Villar J, et al. Association Between Administration of Systemic Corticosteroids and Mortality Among Critically Ill Patients With COVID-19: A Meta-analysis. JAMA. 2020;324(13):1330-41.

19. Van Paassen J, Vos JS, Hoekstra EM, Neumann KMI, Boot PC, Arbous SM. Corticosteroid use in COVID-19 patients: a systematic review and meta-analysis on clinical outcomes. Crit Care. 2020;24(1):696.

20. Granholm A, Munch MW, Myatra SN, Vijayaraghavan BKT, Cronhjort M, Wahlin RR, et al. Dexamethasone 12 mg versus 6 mg for patients with COVID-19 and severe hypoxaemia: a pre-planned, secondary Bayesian analysis of the COVID STEROID 2 trial. Intensive Care Med. 2022;48(1):45-55.

21 Pinzon MA, Ortiz S, Holguin H, Betancur JF, Cardona Arango D, Laniado H, et al. Dexamethasone vs methylprednisolone high dose for Covid-19 pneumonia. PLoS One. 2021;16(5):e0252057.doi.org/10.1371/journal.pone.0252057

22 Ranjbar K, Moghadami M, Mirahmadizadeh A, Fallahi MJ, Khaloo V, Shahriarirad R, et al. Methylprednisolone or dexamethasone, which one is superior corticosteroid in the treatment of hospitalized COVID-19 patients: a triple-blinded randomized controlled trial. BMC Infect Dis. 2021;21(1):337.

23. Hong S, Wang H, Li S, Liu J, Qiao L. A systematic review and meta-analysis of glucocorticoids treatment in severe COVID-19: methylprednisolone versus dexamethasone. BMC Infect Dis. 2023;23(1):290.

24 Tan RSJ, Ng KT, Xin CE, Atan R, Yunos NM, Hasan MS. High-Dose versus Low-Dose Corticosteroids in COVID-19 Patients: a Systematic Review and Meta-analysis. J Cardiothorac Vasc Anesth. 2022;36(9):3576-86.

25. Batirel A, Demirhan R, Eser N, Korlu E, Tezcan ME. Pulse steroid treatment for hospitalized adults with COVID-19. Turk J Med Sci. 2021;51(5):2248-55.

26. Khokher W, Beran A, Iftikhar S, Malhas SE, Srour O, Mhanna M, et al. Pulse versus nonpulse steroid regimens in patients with coronavirus disease 2019: A systematic review and meta-analysis. J Med Virol. 2022;94(9):4125-37.

27 Mohanty RR, Biswa Mohan P, Meher BR. Effectiveness of pulse dose methyl prednisolone in management of COVID 19: A systematic review and meta-analysis of observational studies. J Pharm Pharm Sci. 2022;25:110-23.

28. Force ADT, Ranieri VM, Rubenfeld GD, Thompson BT, Ferguson ND, Caldwell E, et al. Acute respiratory distress syndrome: the Berlin Definition. JAMA. 2012;307(23):2526-33.

29   Grasselli G, Calfee CS, Camporota L, Poole D, Amato MBP, Antonelli M, et al. ESICM guidelines on acute respiratory distress syndrome: definition, phenotyping and respiratory support strategies. Intensive Care Med. 2023;49(7):727-59.

30   Le Gall JR, Lemeshow S, Saulnier F. A new Simplified Acute Physiology Score (SAPS II) based on a European/North American multicenter study. JAMA. 1993;270(24):2957-63.

31   Knaus WA, Draper EA, Wagner DP, Zimmerman JE. APACHE II: a severity of disease classification system. Crit Care Med. 1985;13(10):818-29.

32   Vincent JL, Moreno R, Takala J, Willatts S, De Mendonca A, Bruining H, et al. The SOFA (Sepsis-related Organ Failure Assessment) score to describe organ dysfunction/failure. On behalf of the Working Group on Sepsis-Related Problems of the European Society of Intensive Care Medicine. Intensive Care Med. 1996;22(7):707-10.

33   Bonny V, Maillard A, Mousseaux C, Placais L, Richier Q. [COVID-19: Pathogenesis of a multi-faceted disease]. Rev Med Interne. 2020;41(6):375-89.

34   Jin Y, Yang H, Ji W, Wu W, Chen S, Zhang W, et al. Virology, Epidemiology, Pathogenesis, and Control of COVID-19. Viruses. 2020;12(4).

35   Lamers MM, Beumer J, van der Vaart J, Knoops K, Puschhof J, Breugem TI, et al. SARS-CoV-2 productively infects human gut enterocytes. Science. 2020;369(6499):50-4.

36   Ling Y, Xu SB, Lin YX, Tian D, Zhu ZQ, Dai FH, et al. Persistence and clearance of viral RNA in 2019 novel coronavirus disease rehabilitation patients. Chin Med J (Engl). 2020;133(9):1039-43.

37.   Wu C, Chen X, Cai Y, Xia J, Zhou X, Xu S, et al. Risk Factors Associated With Acute Respiratory Distress Syndrome and Death in Patients With Coronavirus Disease 2019 Pneumonia in Wuhan, China. JAMA Intern Med. 2020;180(7):934-43.

38   Richardson S, Hirsch JS, Narasimhan M, Crawford JM, McGinn T, Davidson KW, et al. Presenting Characteristics, Comorbidities, and Outcomes Among 5700 Patients Hospitalized With COVID-19 in the New York City Area. JAMA. 2020;323(20):2052-9.

39   Changeux JP, Amoura Z, Rey FA, Miyara M. A nicotinic hypothesis for Covid-19 with preventive and therapeutic implications. C R Biol. 2020;343(1):33-9.

40   Li YC, Bai WZ, Hashikawa T. Response to Commentary on "The neuroinvasive potential of SARS-CoV-2 may play a role in the respiratory failure of COVID-19 patients". J Med Virol. 2020;92(7):707-9.

41   Arentz M, Yim E, Klaff L, Lokhandwala S, Riedo FX, Chong M, et al. Characteristics and Outcomes of 21 Critically Ill Patients With COVID-19 in Washington State. JAMA. 2020;323(16):1612-4.

42.   Wang D, Hu B, Hu C, Zhu F, Liu X, Zhang J, et al. Clinical Characteristics of 138 Hospitalized Patients With 2019 Novel Coronavirus-Infected Pneumonia in Wuhan, China. JAMA. 2020;323(11):1061-9.

43   Zhou F, Yu T, Du R, Fan G, Liu Y, Liu Z, et al. Clinical course and risk factors for mortality of adult inpatients with COVID-19 in Wuhan, China: a retrospective cohort study. Lancet. 2020;395(10229):1054-62.

44   Shi S, Qin M, Shen B, Cai Y, Liu T, Yang F, et al. Association of Cardiac Injury With Mortality in Hospitalized Patients With COVID-19 in Wuhan, China. JAMA Cardiol. 2020;5(7):802-10.

45   Fox SE, Akmatbekov A, Harbert JL, Li G, Quincy Brown J, Vander Heide RS. Pulmonary and cardiac pathology in African American patients with COVID-19: an autopsy series from New Orleans. Lancet Respir Med. 2020;8(7):681-6.

46   Nelson BC, Laracy J, Shoucri S, Dietz D, Zucker J, Patel N, et al. Clinical Outcomes Associated With Methylprednisolone in Mechanically Ventilated Patients With COVID-19. Clin Infect Dis. 2021 May 4;72(9):e367-e372. doi:10.1093/cid/ciaa1163. PMID: 32772069; PMCID: PMC7454332.

47   Lu X, Chen T, Wang Y, Wang J, Yan F. Adjuvant corticosteroid therapy for critically ill patients with COVID-19. Crit Care. 2020;24(1):241.

48.   Bani-Sadr F, Hentzien M, Pascard M, N'Guyen Y, Servettaz A, Andreoletti L, et al. Corticosteroid therapy for patients with COVID-19 pneumonia: a before-after study. Int J Antimicrob Agents. 2020;56(2):106077.doi.org/10.1016/j.ijantimicag.2020.106077

49   Fadel R, Morrison AR, Vahia A, Smith ZR, Chaudhry Z, Bhargava P, et al. Early Short-Course Corticosteroids in Hospitalized Patients With COVID-19. Clin Infect Dis. 2020;71(16):2114-20.

50   Fernandez-Cruz A, Ruiz-Antoran B, Munoz-Gomez A, Sancho-Lopez A, Mills-Sanchez P, Centeno-Soto GA, et al. A Retrospective Controlled Cohort Study of the Impact of Glucocorticoid Treatment in SARS-CoV-2 Infection Mortality. Antimicrob Agents Chemother. 2020;64(9).

51   Gong Y, Guan L, Jin Z, Chen S, Xiang G, Gao B. Effects of methylprednisolone use on viral genomic nucleic acid negative conversion and CT imaging lesion absorption in COVID-19 patients under 50 years old. J Med Virol. 2020;92(11):2551-5.

52   Hu Y, Wang T, Hu Z, Wang X, Zhang Z, Li L, et al. Clinical efficacy of glucocorticoid on the treatment of patients with COVID-19 pneumonia: A single-center experience. Biomed Pharmacother. 2020 Oct;130:110529. doi:10.1016/j.biopha.2020.110529. Epub 2020 Jul 28. PMID: 32736237; PMCID: PMC7386262.

53   Li Y, Zhou X, Li T, Chan S, Yu Y, Ai JW, et al. Corticosteroid prevents COVID-19 progression within its therapeutic window: a multicentre, proof-of-concept, observational study. Emerg Microbes Infect. 2020;9(1):1869-77.

54   Ma Y, Zeng H, Zhan Z, Lu H, Zeng Z, He C, et al. Corticosteroid Use in the Treatment of COVID-19: A Multicenter Retrospective Study in Hunan, China. Front Pharmacol. 2020;11:1198.

55   Majmundar M, Kansara T, Lenik JM, Park H, Ghosh K, Doshi R, et al (2020) Efficacy of corticosteroids in non-intensive care unit patients with COVID-19 pneumonia from the New York Metropolitan region . PLoS ONE 15(9): e0238827. https://doi.org/10.1371/journal.pone.0238827

56   Mikulska M, Nicolini LA, Signori A, Di Biagio A, Sepulcri C, Russo C, et al. Tocilizumab and steroid treatment in patients with COVID-19 pneumonia. PLoS One . 2020 Aug 20;15(8):e0237831. doi: 10.1371/journal.pone.0237831. PMID: 32817707; PMCID: PMC7440633.

57   Salton F, Confalonieri P, Meduri GU, Santus P, Harari S, Scala R, et al. Prolonged Low-Dose Methylprednisolone in Patients With Severe COVID-19 Pneumonia. Open Forum Infect Dis. 2020 Sep 12;7(10):ofaa421. doi: 10.1093/ofid/ofaa421. PMID: 33072814; PMCID: PMC7543560.

58   Booth CM, Matukas LM, Tomlinson GA, Rachlis AR, Rose DB, Dwosh HA, et al. Clinical features and short-term outcomes of 144 patients with SARS in the greater Toronto area. JAMA. 2003;289(21):2801-9.

59   Chen CY, Lee CH, Liu CY, Wang JH, Wang LM, Perng RP. Clinical features and outcomes of severe acute respiratory syndrome and predictive factors for acute respiratory distress syndrome. J Chin Med Assoc. 2005;68(1):4-10.

60   Peiris JS, Chu CM, Cheng VC, Chan KS, Hung IF, Poon LL, et al. Clinical progression and viral load in a community outbreak of coronavirus-associated SARS pneumonia: a prospective study. Lancet. 2003;361(9371):1767-72.

61   Sung JJ, Wu A, Joynt GM, Yuen KY, Lee N, Chan PK, et al. Severe acute respiratory syndrome: report of treatment and outcome after a major outbreak. Thorax. 2004;59(5):414-20.

62.   Hasan SS, Capstick T, Ahmed R, Kow CS, Mazhar F, Merchant HA, et al. Mortality in COVID-19 patients with acute respiratory distress syndrome and corticosteroids use: a systematic review and meta-analysis. Expert Rev Respir Med. 2020;14(11):1149-63.

63   Papazian L, Aubron C, Brochard L, Chiche JD, Combes A, Dreyfuss D, et al. Formal guidelines: management of acute respiratory distress syndrome. Ann Intensive Care. 2019;9(1):69.

APPENDIX S

APPENDICES

Appendix 1: SAPS II

Table 3.—SAPS II Scoring Sheet*

Variable	Points: 26	13	12	11	9	7	6	5	4	3	2	0
Age, y												<40
Heart rate, beats/min				<40							40-69	70-119
Systolic BP, mm Hg		<70						70-99				100-199
Body temperature, °C (°F)												<39° (<102.2°)
Only if ventilated or continuous pulmonary artery pressure Pao$_2$, mm Hg/Fio$_2$				<100	100-199		≥200					
Pao$_2$, kPa/Fio$_2$				<13.3	13.3-26.5		≥26.6					
Urinary output, L/d				<0.500					0.500-0.999			≥1.000
Serum urea level, mmol/L (g/L) or serum urea nitrogen level, mg/dL												<10.0 (<0.60) <28
WBC count (10³/cu mm)			<1.0									1.0-19.9
Serum potassium, mmol/d										<3.0		3.0-4.9
Serum sodium level, mmol/L								<125				125-144
Serum bicarbonate level, mEq/L							<15			15-19		≥20
Bilirubin level, µmol/L (mg/dL)												<68.4 (<4.0)
Glasgow Coma Score	<6	6-8				9-10		11-13				14-15
Chronic diseases												
Type of admission												Scheduled surgical
Sum of points												

Table 4.—Variables and Definitions for SAPS II*

Variable	Definition
Age	Use the patient's age (in years) at last birthday
Heart rate	Use the worst value in 24 hours, either low or high heart rate; if it varied from cardiac arrest (11 points) to extreme tachycardia (7 points), assign 11 points
Systolic blood pressure	Use the same method as for heart rate; eg, if it varied from 60 mm Hg to 205 mm Hg, assign 13 points
Body temperature	Use the highest temperature in degrees Centigrade or Fahrenheit
Pao$_2$/Fio$_2$ ratio	If ventilated or continuous pulmonary artery pressure, use the lowest value of the ratio
Urinary output	If the patient is in the intensive care unit for less than 24 hours, make the calculation for 24 hours; eg, 1 L in 8 hours = 3 L in 24 hours
Serum urea or serum urea nitrogen level	Use the highest value in mmol/L or g/L for serum urea, in mg/dL for serum urea nitrogen
WBC count	Use the worst (high or low) WBC count according to the scoring sheet
Serum potassium level	Use the worst (high or low) value in mmol/L, according to the scoring sheet
Serum sodium level	Use the worst (high or low) value in mmol/L, according to the scoring sheet
Serum bicarbonate level	Use the lowest value in mEq/L
Bilirubin level	Use the highest value in µmol/L or mg/dL
Glasgow Coma Score	Use the lowest value; if the patient is sedated, record the estimated Glasgow Coma Score before sedation
Type of admission	Unscheduled surgical,† scheduled surgical,‡ or medical§
AIDS	Yes, if HIV-positive with clinical complications such as *Pneumocystis carinii* pneumonia, Kaposi's sarcoma, lymphoma, tuberculosis, or toxoplasma infection
Hematologic malignancy	Yes, if lymphoma, acute leukemia, or multiple myeloma
Metastatic cancer	Yes, if proven metastasis by surgery, computed tomographic scan, or any other method

The APACHE II Severity of Disease Classification System

Physiologic Variable	+4	+3	+2	+1	0	+1	+2	+3	+4
Temperature - rectal (°C)	≥41	39-40.9		38.5-38.9	36-38.4	34-35.9	32-33.9	30-31.9	≤29.9
Mean Arterial Pressure (mm Hg)	≥160	130-159	110-129		70-109		50-69		≤49
Heart Rate	≥180	140-179	110-139		70-109		55-69	40-54	≤39
Respiratory Rate (nonventilated or ventilated)	≥50	35-49		25-34	12-24	10-11	6-9		≤5
Oxygenation (mmHg) a. FiO_2 > 0,5 use A-aDO_2 b. FiO_2 < 0,5 use PaO_2	a: ≥500 b:	350-499	200-349		a: <200 b: > 70	61-70		55-60	<55
Arterial pH	≥7.7	7.6-7.69		7.5-7.59	7.33-7.49		7.25-7.32	7.15-7.24	<7.15
Serum Sodium (mmol/l)	≥180	160-179	155-159	150-154	130-149		120-129	111-119	≤110
Serum Potassium (mmol/l)	≥7	6-6.9		5.5-5.9	3.5-5.4	3-3.4	2.5-2.9		<2.5
Serum Creatinine (mg/dl, Double point score for acute renal failure)	≥3.5	2-3.4	1.5-1.9		0.6-1.4		<0.6		
Hematocrit (%)	≥60		50-59.9	46-49.9	30-45.9		20-29.9		<20
White Blood Count (in 1000/mm³)	≥40		20-39.9	15-19.9	3-14.9		1-2.9		<1
Glasgow-Coma-Scale (GCS)	Score = 15 minus actual GCS								
Serum HCO_3 (venous, mmol/l, use if no ABGs)	≥52	41-51.9		32-40.9	22-31.9		18-21.9	15-17.9	<15
A = Total Acute Physiology Score APS	Sum of the 12 individual variable points								

B = Age Points	C = Chronic Health Points
≤44 years — 0 points 45-54 years — 2 points 55-64 years — 3 points 65-74 years — 5 points ≥75 years — 6 points	If the patient has a history of severe organ system insufficiency or is immunocompromised assign points as follows: a. For nonoperative or emergency postoperative patients – 5 points b. For elective postoperative patients – 2 points

APACHE II Score = Sum of A (APS points) + B (Age points) + C (Chronic Health points)

(From: Knaus WA, Draper EA, Wagner DP, Zimmerman JE. APACHE II: a severity of disease classification system. Crit Care Med 1985;13(10):818-29)

Appendix 3: SOFA Score

	Score				
Système	0	1	2	3	4
Respiration PaO2/FiO2, mmHg (kPa)	≥ 400 (53,3)	<400 (53,3)	< 300 (40)	<200 (26,7) avec soutien ventilatoire	<100 (13,3) avec soutien ventilatoire
Coagulation Plaquettes, x10^3/µl	≥ 150	< 150	<100	< 50	< 20
Foie Bilirubine, µmol/l (mg/dl)	<1,2 (20)	1,2-1,9 (20-32)	2,0-5,9 (33-101)	6,0-11,9 (102-204)	>12,0 (204)
Cardiovasculaire	PAM ≥ 70 mmHg	PAM < 70 mmHg	Dopamine < 5 ou dobutamine (toute dose)*	Dopamine 5,1-15 ou adrénaline ≤ 0,1 ou noradrénaline ≤ 0,1*	Dopamine <15 ou adrénaline >0,1 ou noradrénaline >0,1*
Système nerveux central Glasgow Coma Scale	15	13-14	10-12	6-9	<6
Rénal Créatinine, µmol/l (mg/dl) Diurèse, ml/j	<1,2 (110)	1,2-1,9 (110-170)	2,0-3,4 (171-299)	3,5-4,9 (300-400) <500	>5 (440) <200

PaO2: partial pressure of oxygen; FiO2: fraction of inspired oxygen; MAP: mean arterial pressure.

* catecholamine doses are given in µg/kg/min

Summary

Méduri protocol and COVID19 pneumonia: Factors in therapeutic failure

Summary

SARS-CoV-2 causes ARDS, a cytokine storm and excessive inflammation... High-dose corticosteroid therapy may be indicated in patients who develop pulmonary fibrosis. The aim of the study was to identify the factors leading to failure of high-dose corticosteroid therapy according to the Meduri protocol. This prospective cohort study was conducted in the intensive care unit of the Taher Sfar Hospital in Mahdia. All patients hospitalised with SARS-CoV-2 pneumonia received methylprednisolone 2 mg/kg/d in tapering doses over one month. Out of 178 patients, treatment success was 33.7%, with a mortality rate of 61%. In multivariate analysis, SAPS II score (OR=0.938, CI95% [0.895-0.982], p=0.007) and use of NIV (OR=0.416, CI95% [0.187-0.925], p=0.031) were independently associated with failure. The SAPS II threshold was 23.5 with a sensitivity of 75%, a specificity of 61%, a positive predictive value of 54.55%, a negative predictive value of 79.46% and an area under the curve of 0.724. In conclusion, the SAPS II score and the use of NIV are factors in failure.

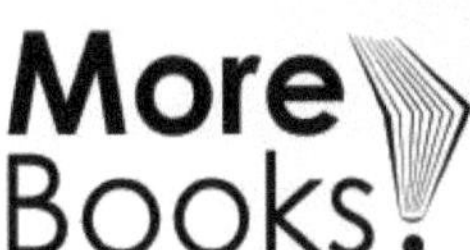

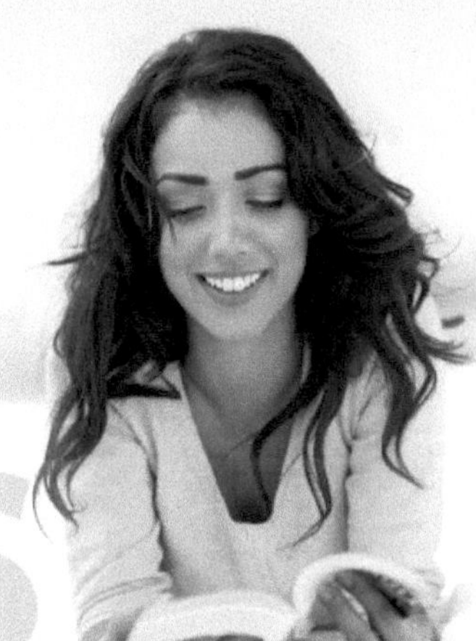

I want morebooks!

Buy your books fast and straightforward online - at one of world's fastest growing online book stores! Environmentally sound due to Print-on-Demand technologies.

Buy your books online at
www.morebooks.shop

Kaufen Sie Ihre Bücher schnell und unkompliziert online – auf einer der am schnellsten wachsenden Buchhandelsplattformen weltweit! Dank Print-On-Demand umwelt- und ressourcenschonend produziert.

Bücher schneller online kaufen
www.morebooks.shop

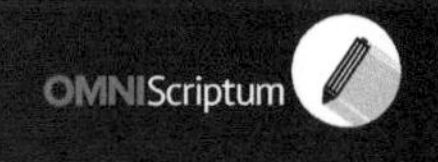

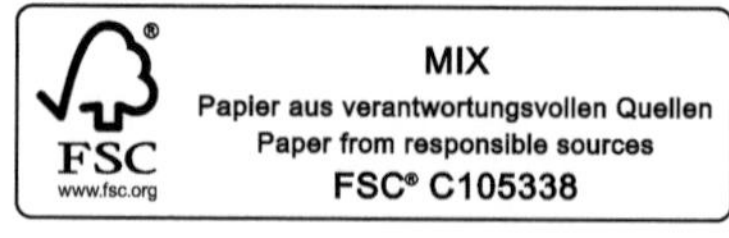

Printed by Books on Demand GmbH, Norderstedt / Germany